Susie & Herman

Susie
& Herman

A Story of Love and Caregiving

L. B. SMITH

Health Communications, Inc.
Deerfield Beach, Florida

www.hci-online.com

Library of Congress Cataloging-in-Publication Data

Smith, L. B., date.
    Susie & Herman : a story of love and caregiving / L. B. Smith.
      p.   cm.
    ISBN 1-55874-957-8
    1. Smith, L. B., 1939-.   2. Caregivers—United States—
Biography.   3. Aged—Care—United States.   4. Dementia—
Patients—Care—United States.   I. Title: Susie and Herman.
II. Title.

HV1461 .S557 2002
365.1'9683—dc21
[B]

2001051639

HCI, its Logos and Marks are trademarks of Health Communications,
Inc.

Publisher: Health Communications, Inc.
               3201 S.W. 15th Street
               Deerfield Beach, FL 33442-8190

Cover and inside book design by Lawna Patterson Oldfield
Cover photo ©PhotoDisc

To Emil and Susie,
my parents, whose love, guidance,
patience and example led me
to become the caregiver
I became.

Contents

ACKNOWLEDGMENTS

It all started with Gary Seidler listening to the stories my wife Suzanne would tell him about my almost-daily experiences looking after Mom and Herman. Being the journalist and publisher that he is, he began encouraging me to put these experiences into written form. In other words, write a book.

It took three years and the expert help of Steve Ricci—writer, editor and a man with the patience required to correct my English—to put the words in the proper order and even rewrite entire pages. Without Steve's help, I couldn't have gotten the story told.

During the writing of this book (we were also living it in real time), many things happened: We lost my mother, who was a wonderful mother, wife, grandmother and great-grandmother; and just six months ago, we lost Herman. A true ending to the story. I always had the support of my wonderful wife, Suzanne, who saw me through all the trying times, both day and night. She would wait up for me on those late-night returns from the hospital ER or from the late-night emergencies that fortunately did not end up in the ER.

I also want to thank my daughter, Deanna Insua, who spent some long days and evenings in the hospital and at my mom's apartment visiting. She would bring her sons to visit, too. (The boys were not eager to visit Great-Grandma very often—but, that's boys.) My daughter Deborah Tojeiro also helped Mom by bringing her to the rehab center to visit Herman, taking her grocery shopping or just coming to visit with her own daughter, Ashlie. My daughter, Janee Womack, always volunteered her time, her car and herself to run errands of all sorts. In other words, it was a family effort. And without them I would have been hard-pressed to accomplish this monumental task of being a caregiver.

Sadly, my son, David Smith, lives in Dallas and would only see Grandma when he flew in to our area (he is a pilot), but she always had a special place in her heart for him, her first grandchild.

I want to thank a very important person, Pam Traeger, who spent seven days a week, twenty-four hours a day taking care of Herman and Susie. She made sure that they ate, were bathed daily and dressed in clean clothes. In short, she cared for them as though they were her own family. We all truly love Pam for her dedication, caring, skill and, most of all, her untiring efforts to ensure their comfort and safety. Thank you, Pam, thank you!!!!

Also, thank you, Dr. Jeffrey Levy, their doctor, who was always there for them at the ER, or on the phone with Pam or myself, at any time.

Last, thanks to Peter Vegso, who read the book and decided to publish it. This book is a bit out of character for Health Communications, but Peter elected to publish it anyhow. Thank you again, Peter.

FOREWORD

Roses in December

This is a personal story. This is a story of our times.

The dementias are a group of brain disorders that represent one of the greatest public-health challenges of the coming generation. The vicissitudes of dealing with dementia from an individual and a societal perspective exact enormous social, personal and economic costs. L. B. Smith has provided a humane, loving and insightful lens that exposes an increasingly common problem that will affect virtually every family at some level. His personal account describes the anguish, joys, anxiety and daily fear of catastrophe that characterize the lives of caregivers. With warmth and compassion, he illustrates the "payback" for a lifetime of support and nurturing that he received from his caregivers, now his charges. Through this account, we see the need to balance risk with dignity, respect for independence and quality of life. The list of concerns is endless: driving, fire, wandering, financial exploitation and more.

As a geriatric psychiatrist involved in the development of services, training and research into the psychiatric disorders of late life, I have seen firsthand that caregivers are one of the greatest assets that our society possesses, providing support that would otherwise fall to the state. The informal caregiver is a versatile individual indeed, functioning as counselor/advisor, case manager, banker, nurse's aide, advocate, ingenious problem solver and chauffeur (especially to doctors' offices), to name just a few of the cameo roles that these valuable individuals must play.

At the same time, finding formal caregivers who supplement the role of family and friends is equally important; these angels are highly valued and appreciated.

The postscripts throughout the book provide insights into the dynamics of caregiving as role reversals and the stressors of caregiving reprise earlier memories, experiences and conflicts. L. B. Smith shows at a very personal level the effects of caregiving on health and its impact on his own attitudes about possible dependency in the future. We see both humor and pathos in the simultaneous observation of a changing organism and participation in a changing relationship. The disturbed sleep, interrupted meals, missed business meetings and disrupted holidays are part and parcel of the selfless task of caregiving. The telephone is both a blessing and a torment. The caregiver deals with repetitiveness, suspiciousness, paranoid thinking, accusations of stealing, hoarding and highly embarrassing moments. To all of this, L. B. Smith reveals his selfless sacrifice to those he truly loves and cares for. The cost is not insignificant but the rewards and gratification are substantial, looking back on the fulfillment of an important role.

This is an important book for caregivers to share and compare personal experiences, both for those of us who have been through, or are going through, similar experiences and for a future generation who will do well to gird themselves for the challenge that lies ahead. Both for himself and for all of us, L. B. Smith has encapsulated the memories of a difficult but important role that most of us will face at some stage.

God gave us memories so we could have roses in December. So, too, the final memories of these important relationships will sustain Mr. Smith and his readers.

KENNETH I. SHULMAN
Professor of Psychiatry
University of Toronto

INTRODUCTION

The Memoirs of a Caregiver

In assessing the needs of the elderly, many people mistakenly compare them to children. For children, the future is lit by the bright promise of what lies ahead. For the dependent elderly, the future is obscured by uncertainty and fear.

Children are learning what they don't yet know; many elderly people, however, are forgetting what they always knew. They are fighting a war of attrition, with bodies slowly becoming insufficient for the demands of everyday activities; with minds gradually becoming unable to decipher a complex and intolerant world that grows more baffling each day.

As they grow, children use their newfound knowledge to gain confidence and self-reliance. The process is reversed when elderly people who can no longer sustain their own care must surrender control of their circumstances to someone else—an agonizing decision for those who have supported themselves and others for their entire lives. Often, they turn to their adult children, who have raised (or may still be raising) families of their own.

The past six years of my life have been consumed by the ponderous task of caring for my ninety-two-year-old mother, Susie, and her husband, Herman. It was, without a doubt, the most difficult and stressful endeavor of my life. With few other relatives or family friends to share the burden, balancing the responsibilities of a career, a home and children make caregiving a truly maddening, frustrating, exhausting experience. I don't imagine that someone who has never assumed the care of a dependent person can fully comprehend the toll such an undertaking exacts on both the mind and the body.

I've learned that getting through the adversities depends on two things: The first is a sense of humor. Approaching the care of a dependent person necessarily involves, at best, inconvenience, and, at worst, pain. How you choose to deal with these trials will directly determine how deeply it affects you and to what degree your life is altered by it. The second is empathy. Caring for someone with special needs, especially the elderly, requires the caregiver to accept that, in the future, he or she may be in the same situation. Knowing that you may one day find yourself traveling in a car with no idea how you got there or where you're going is a stark but effective reminder that the degree to which we depend on others now will be magnified tenfold when our mental or physical capacities are compromised.

For the caregiver, the struggle to care for those who cannot sustain themselves is one without victories. The constant phone calls, troubles with nurses and aides, pointless bickering, missed appointments and frustrating memory loss can easily push even the most serene of us to the

brink of rage. Surviving the implicit discourage-
ment and despondency requires an ability to
treat serious subjects lightly and an awareness
that each of us, regardless of our current circumstances, might one day feel as equally alone,
afraid and bewildered.

For many caregivers, finding humor in calamity
is the most difficult virtue to achieve. While we
may feel enraged, confounded, depressed, discour-
aged, fatigued, even wounded at times, the people
to whom we are devoting our time, energy, love
and money sometimes can barely comprehend
what is going on around them, let alone the sacrifices being made on their behalf. They seem to
live in a parallel universe, where the things that
are important to us are trivial to them, and what
is absurd to us is monumental to them.

This book is intended for those caregivers—
adults with jobs, families, responsibilities and
commitments who have dedicated themselves to
caring for their elderly parents or other dependent family members. This is not a how-to book or
a manual on the care and feeding of the elderly. It

is not offered as professional advice, counsel or coaching for the caregiver. Certainly, it is not meant to mock, demean or lampoon the failings of the elderly.

It is, instead, a memoir of the ordeals and adventures I've encountered in caring for Susie and Herman—incidents similar to those that other caregivers face daily. I also offer a few suggestions on coping strategies that worked for me.

Throughout my life, I've been given all kinds of advice, some of it fairly good, some of it not so good, some of it downright stupid. The best advice I ever received was from my mother. When your mother gives you advice, there's no hidden meaning in it, only concern for what is in your best interest. It wasn't an earth-shaking revelation, just something that stuck with me because it is important yet simple. She said, "Be honest with yourself. You have to be honest with yourself before you can find happiness and figure out who and what you want to be and what you want out of life." That means accepting who you are and what you are and coming to terms with that before you can expect certain things from other people.

In caring for Susie and Herman, I tried to keep this principle in mind. I struggled to remember that if I deny the anger, frustration and sadness that were natural parts of the task I had undertaken, then I was not being honest with myself. As a result, the negative effects of those feelings would intensify and harden into resentment, pessimism and contempt. Instead, I tried to accept the feelings as they came and understand that there was humor in the absurdity, the contradictions, the contentiousness and the disintegration. In doing so, my perspective changed and I learned that, above all, caregiving is about dignity. It is about having the patience, compassion and empathy to give someone the benefit of your caring in the knowledge that you, in turn, may someday rely on the same qualities in another person.

I've tried to pass my mother's wisdom on to my children when I give them advice. Through openness and honesty, I've encouraged them to seek their own answers and their own spiritual guidance. As her wisdom helped me make caregiving decisions for her, I hope that by passing it on to my children, I can help them do the same if they are ever faced with the same choices regarding my care.

All of us face the prospect of someday becoming dependent on another person for our safety and well-being. By lighting a candle today, we can curse the darkness tomorrow.

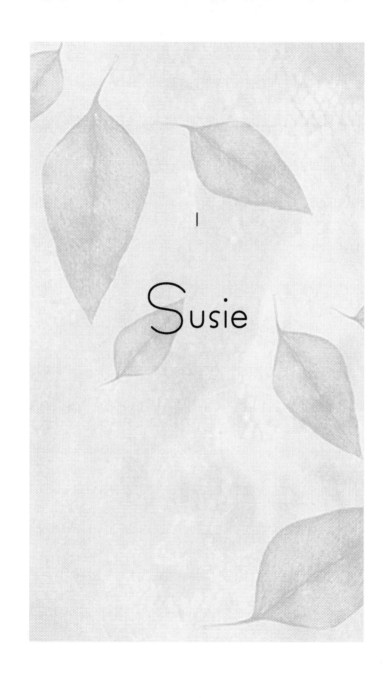

I

Susie

My mother, Susie, was a kind, sweet and personable woman who was liked by everyone she knew. She was born in Bayreuth, Germany, on September 26, 1906, the older of two girls. Her father was a liquor distributor and her mother was a homemaker. Because of the limited scope of public schools at the time, her father sent Susie to a private Catholic school. After graduating high school, she attended university for two years, which was rare for women at that time.

In 1929, Susie married Emil Schmidt, whose family owned a slaughterhouse and a meat-packing plant. In 1933, due to the radically changing economic and sociologic ideals in Germany, they decided to emigrate to the

United States, specifically New York City.

Susie's relationship with her husband was loving and respectful. As they worked and prospered in America, economic and political turmoil was on the rise in Germany. Because of the anti-German sentiment in America at the outbreak of World War II, they changed their name from Schmidt to Smith. They did this, in part, to protect me, their only child.

When I was a toddler, the family moved to the Bronx, where they would remain for many years. Despite the troubles in their homeland, the family prospered in America and built comfortable lives. Shortly before the United States entered the war, the Smiths brought Susie's parents, sister and brother-in-law to America and helped them establish themselves.

My father worked extremely hard in the wholesale meat business, rising at 4:00 A.M. and returning each day in the late afternoon. When I was a teenager, I could never understand why my friends always got to eat the "good stuff," like hamburgers and hot dogs, while we were always eating steak, veal and pork chops. I remember telling Mom that I hated eating at our house and wanted to eat at my friends' homes because they had better food. She would try to explain that, because my father was in the wholesale meat business, he could bring home the best cuts of meat, so much in fact, that the freezer would be overflowing and he would give away some to the neighbors. While my friends were eating ground beef, I was eating the finest cuts of meat in New York and didn't even know it.

Susie was also a remarkably hard worker. In 1951, she began working at Bloomingdale's in New York City and stayed with the company for thirty-five years. When she retired in 1986 at eighty years of age, I believe she had achieved the second-highest seniority at the company. For the last ten years of her time there, she worked four hours a day, two or three days a week, just so she could feel useful.

But my parents knew that life was about more than work. As teenagers, we often looked upon as strange or weird some of the things our parents did. My parents loved getting together with friends and neighbors for evenings of eating and drinking. Invariably, the group would gather around the piano. One of their best friends was a piano player who, despite an unfortunate accident that cost him the middle two fingers of his left hand, could still manage to play quite well. Another neighbor played the violin, and it wasn't long before the house was rocking with 1930s and 1940s dance music. To my chagrin, they often tried to engage me in the merriment— not something a teenager looks forward to doing. I sometimes was successful in my attempts to hide, and other times I wasn't as lucky. Today, I can see why my own kids, when they were in their teens, disappeared when my wife and I gave a party.

In 1963, my father was diagnosed with advanced colon cancer. In the early 1960s, with medical science lacking today's advanced technology, this diagnosis was a virtual death sentence. Although surgery helped him bounce back a bit, it wasn't enough. My first wife and I were in her hometown of Fort Worth, Texas, to visit her father in the hospital recovering from a heart attack when we received a telegram notifying us that my father had relapsed.

We got the first flight we could back to New York. I made it to the hospital with only minutes to spare. When I saw my father, he recognized me and talked to me for a few minutes, clearly happy to see me. He passed away while holding my hand.

His death was one of the biggest sorrows in my life. I was glad that I reached him before he died, but I was very much saddened that I had so little time to spend with him before his passing. My father's death was especially tragic in that his life was cut short at the age of fifty-six. He'd spent most of his life working, usually twelve to fourteen hours a day, establishing his own business and working away at it. His schedule did not allow us much time to spend together. I remember being jealous of my friends whose fathers had more time to devote to them. My mother used to say that my father was working that hard for me.

At the time I didn't understand, but having since become both a father and a grandfather, my father's sacrifices mean much more to me.

Mom continued on after Emil's death, working, visiting friends and seeing her family. Traveling was among her favorite activities, and she did it often. She moved back to Manhattan and became friends with a neighbor named Erna, who was also a widow and lived in the same building. Together, they would travel to Europe each summer, especially to their favorite place, Merano, in northern Italy.

Mom was also a superb cook, who would spend days in the kitchen baking cookies and pies from scratch. Her scrumptious Christmas cookies were in such demand in our family that she made enough to last three or four months, and still had to hide them all over the house so they wouldn't be devoured.

Her sense of direction was a wholly different story. Despite her exceptional knowledge of New York City, outside the borough of Manhattan she was like a baby bird out of its nest. Once, on a business trip to the New York area, I stayed with Mom to take advantage of some good home cooking. During my stay, we were invited to visit my cousin who lived in New Jersey. Although I'd only been there once, she'd been there at least a hundred times. And yet, once we were out of the Lincoln Tunnel, she had no idea where we were going and we drove aimlessly for hours. Because she had become dependent on the city's public transportation, driving was never an option for Susie.

As she entered her eighties, Susie began having trouble with the rigors of life in the cold and sometimes dangerous atmosphere of New York; she'd been robbed several times. Eventually, I talked her into moving to South Florida, where I had been living for about twenty-five years. Although she missed New York, she accepted that it was time for an easier and safer lifestyle closer to those who could care for her.

By 1993, Susie was becoming forgetful. She would put food on the stove and forget it was there. Going to the supermarket was frightening for her because she didn't drive, and she would become confused riding the bus and forget her way home. It was time to find a retirement facility that would suit Mom and her needs.

Not long after moving into her new retirement facility, she met Herman, the second great love of her life. Herman was a widower, six months Susie's elder, who was known for his cute, charming, flirtatious personality. Herman, like Susie, was also from Germany, and he had retired as the general manager of a nationally known uniform manufacturer. He loved to paint, play chess and listen to opera.

He befriended Susie and invited her to come with him on trips to California and Israel. Six months later, to the shock of our family, Susie announced that Herman had asked her to marry him. The family recommended that they first live together and they did give it a try. However, their traditional values made them feel guilty living in the same apartment unmarried. They persisted in their plans, and we eventually decided that the couple's happiness and peace of mind was the paramount issue. Being married clearly made Susie and Herman feel more connected to each other and at peace with their consciences.

On May 22, 1995, their friends and family gathered for a small ceremony at the facility where Susie and Herman lived to watch two people who had lived a long time declare their love for each other in the waning years of their lives.

As you will see in the coming chapters, their brief life together was a series of highs and lows, happiness and tribulation. They found joy and comfort in having the other always nearby. No matter where they went—walking around the lobby, sitting on the sofa watching television or at each other's bedside at the hospital—they were always holding hands. At the same time, their growing infirmities and diminishing faculties made daily living a challenging and exasperating ordeal for them and for our family.

2

The Cadillac Option

The time had come for my mother to move to the independent-living facility she had selected. We had hoped she'd choose a facility close to our home in Boca Raton so that family visits would be convenient. She had other plans. An old friend of hers lived in a facility in North Miami Beach, some forty miles away, and a former coworker from her days working at Bloomingdale's in New York lived nearby. We readied ourselves for hours of driving congested South Florida highways each time we wanted to visit.

At first the travel was tolerable, but the miles between us seemed to grow in direct relation to the demands placed on my time by family and work responsibilities. Although Mom (who since moving to the facility had met and moved in with Herman) needed my help more than ever, visiting more frequently than two or three times a week was becoming impossible. It was time for a solution. Like a distinguished, experienced barrister arguing an open-and-shut case, I expounded on the burden that traveling such a great distance placed on us, the limited amount of time we had to spend with them, the need to be closer in case of emergency and the added benefit of more visits from grandchildren and great-grandchildren. Calmly, reasonably and logically, I outlined the many benefits for all involved if they would only consider moving to a facility closer to our home. Perry Mason and Matlock would have wept at my performance.

They listened patiently to my arguments and carefully formed their response: "We want to get a car."

Suddenly, I pictured national news reports of a forty-car pileup snarling rush-hour traffic on I-95 because of two nonagenarians driving in the wrong direction down the carpool lane while looking for a Denny's. I imagined myself being arrested and hauled before an enraged judge who would vilify me as the monster who allowed his elderly mother and her husband to operate a motor vehicle on the mean streets of South Florida. Just as they were adjusting the electric-chair straps, I snapped out of my fantasy and realized that I needed to give them another option immediately.

"Taxis," I said cautiously. They were a lot less expensive. You didn't need to worry about high insurance rates, registration fees, oil changes, tires, tune-ups, breakdowns or getting into accidents. Herman responded by flashing his driver's license at me and pointing out the "safe driver" notation. Lacking an alternate defense, I decided to drop the issue in the hopes they'd soon abandon this ridiculous concept. Little was said over the course of the next month. However, on occasion during trips to the doctor's office or the supermarket, my mother would nonchalantly mention how nice it would be if they had their own car and didn't have to rely on us for transportation. I knew that convincing them otherwise would be like trying to bail out the Titanic with a thimble. I immediately changed the subject, hoping the car phase would soon pass.

In my office one day a few weeks later, I received a frantic call from my mother. She said Herman had gone out earlier in the day and had not come back. She had no idea where he'd gone. As I questioned her about the events leading to Herman's departure, my lower jaw almost bounced off the surface of my desk. Apparently, a car sales-man had been to their home four or five hours ear-lier. He had brought a car for them to see. Herman and the salesman went off to close the deal and Herman hadn't been heard from since. Mom had no idea who the salesman was, what dealership he represented or where they had gone.

I hung up immediately and called a friend with the Metro-Dade Police Department. About five minutes later, Mom called again. Herman had returned. I breathed a sigh of relief and awaited the explanation.

Herman had seen a newspaper ad from a local dealer in used cars. He called and told them he'd like a car and had about six thousand dollars to spend. Within the hour, a beaming salesman appeared with a 1989 Sedan de Ville that he thought he might be able to let go for six thousand dollars, and he, Herman and Mom went for a little ride around the block. As would any shrewd consumer trying to strike a bargain by appearing casually disinterested, Mom said, "Let's take it!" They dropped her off at the house and drove to the dealership about five miles away to close the deal.

The papers signed, Herman departed the dealership behind the wheel of his new car and promptly realized he didn't know his exact street address or how to get back home. He spent the better part of the next three hours trying vainly to find his way home, finally paying a cabdriver to lead the way to a familiar street.

After I recovered from the shock of this harrowing news, I immediately set about devising a way to separate them from their vehicle as efficiently and precisely as the dealer had in separating them from their money. They decided they wanted me to see the car for myself and take a ride with them.

At first glance, it was a pretty white car with a red, padded vinyl roof. Closer examination, however, revealed rust along the tops of the door and trunk frames. The mileage was also excessively high. I estimated the car's value at roughly half what they had paid for it and imagined the salesman was doing cartwheels around the dealership while regaling his buddies with stories about the two old codgers who handed him six large and said, "We want a car."

I was distracted again by Herman's cheerful exclamation, "Let's go for a ride," and silently prayed that my life-insurance premiums had been fully paid. He stepped into the car, started the engine and threw it into reverse. He failed to realize, however, that I hadn't gotten in the car yet and was still standing next to the open door, which almost knocked me down when it hit me. I politely declined the ride and told them that, until they bought proper insurance coverage to protect their assets, they could not use the car.

The car dealer had provided Herman only minimum liability insurance on a temporary binder. It would do almost nothing to protect them in the event they caused a serious accident.

Finding insurance for Herman at his advanced age was going to be difficult, if not impossible. Herman and Mom, however, would not be deterred. While we negotiated with the insurance company, they insisted on driving the car around their neighborhood. Herman had no idea where to put the gas nozzle. Nor could he successfully master the complexities of modern self-service pumps. As a result, they drove until the car ran out of gas, at which point they'd call a garage for a fifty-five-dollar tow.

After another outing, he forgot to turn off the car lights and killed the battery. Another fifty-five dollars for a jump start. Herman didn't run the engine for a while and was surprised when he tried to start the car the next day and found the battery still dead. Fifty-five dollars.

The curtain came down on this runaway Burns-and-Allen sketch in the shape of a letter from the insurance company stating that they would not insure Herman without his physician's certification that he was competent to drive. His doctor would not comply, and Herman's driving days were over. I could almost hear the exuberant cheers of joyous fellow motorists drowning out the distressed sighs of despondent tow-truck drivers. That evening, my son-in-law picked up the car and brought it to his house. He washed, waxed and detailed the car, and we sold it about two weeks later for a thirty-five-hundred-dollar loss.

Like Herman and my mom, I had lost a small battle but won a great war. Despite the cost and the potential danger, I had to concede them the right to exert their free will in purchasing the car and attempting to own and operate it. They came to realize that it was not possible—not through my dictating those circumstances to them, but by the trial and error of their own experience.

Of course, I still never managed to convince them to move to Boca Raton.

Postscript

My father worked ten to twelve hours a day, six days a week, and he worked hard. When he wasn't working, one of his big passions was his car. He loved his car above all his other possessions. He loved it like I love boats. When I was able to drive, occasionally he let me use the car, but in return I had to help him wax it on Saturday afternoons. When I got older, I bought my own car and used it to go out on dates and with friends. However, after driving around in my old junker for a while, I was soon coveting Dad's car because it was sharp and shiny, not rusted and run-down like mine. My dad, however, started his job very early in the morning and was reluctant to let me use his car to go out at night because he was afraid that I wouldn't be home by the time he was ready to go to work. Eventually, he relented and gave me the keys, and I always made sure I was back before he left in the morning.

One morning, however, I didn't make it home in time and found him standing there, waiting on the street for me. That was the last time I drove his car for quite a while. Being stranded made my father feel powerless and angry because he was unable to control his own circumstances. Anyone who has ever had their car stolen, experienced a breakdown or even been stuck in a traffic jam knows the frustration of being stranded and helpless. When I saw him standing there waiting for me, I realized that I had robbed him, although briefly and unintentionally, of his control over his own life. It's something I've never forgotten.

Even Americans as old as Herman have lived most of their lives with automobiles. In twenty-first-century America, cars are much more than modes of transportation; they are potent symbols of freedom, expression and movement. Unfortunately, as people age and their faculties diminish, their ability to drive safely also declines. For many elderly people, the loss of their car is the first step in the descent into dependence on others for their day-to-day activities and, therefore, it is usually the hardest thing to surrender.

Herman and Susie clung to the notion that Herman could continue driving, and it became my unpleasant responsibility to convince them otherwise. Once again, I could see my father standing at the side of the road, waiting impatiently and wearing an angry expression that said, "How could you do this to me?" Back then, I did it because I didn't know any better. But for Herman, I did it because by then I *did* know better.

3

Traveling Mercies

For more than twenty years, Mom and her best friend, Erna, traveled throughout the U.S. and Europe. When Mom moved to South Florida in 1987, she and Erna continued their travels; Mom would fly to New York to meet Erna, where they would board a plane for six weeks of fun at some European destination. However, once she moved to the adult congregate living facility, Mom's wanderlust seemed to wane along with her confidence in her ability to travel.

A phase of her life that we thought had ended suddenly started again when, after six months of keeping company with Herman, he invited Mom along as his guest on a three-week trip to Israel. Having Herman on her arm restored her confidence. This was the start of several trips across the country and abroad.

Although it was wonderful to see Mom regain her self-reliance with Herman, their trips were anything but a respite for us. Around the time they were planning what turned out to be their last trip to Israel, Herman's grasp of reality, as well as his ability to successfully control some of his physical functions, had begun to slip considerably. His condition complicated our lives somewhat, but he and Mom seemed utterly unaware of a problem. I tried to talk them out of making the trip, but Herman the Independent insisted that they were going. He called the travel agent, booked the flights and made hotel reservations.

Although departure day was fraught with confusion about packing, passports and pretrip jitters, we helped them get it together and set off for the airport. After much commotion at the ticket counter (they had forgotten about a change of planes in Frankfurt), the intrepid duo left us with a promise to call as soon as they arrived at their destination.

About fifteen hours later, the friends who were to pick them up at the airport in Tel Aviv called to say they never arrived. My imagination immediately kicked into overdrive. Had Herman stumbled into the cockpit while looking for the bathroom and accidentally ejected the pilots into the Atlantic? Perhaps they'd gone to the wrong terminal and were now in a hot-air balloon two thousand feet over the African savannah, scratching their heads and wondering when it was that giraffes started migrating to Israel.

After several frantic calls to Lufthansa Airlines, we discovered that while Mom and Herman were waiting for their connection in Frankfurt, they both fell asleep in the airport and missed the flight. They finally were found by Lufthansa personnel, who babysat them until they were put on another flight and arrived in Israel safe and sound. Their friends found them and took them to the hotel.

Tired of waiting for their call to say they'd arrived safely, I tried in vain to reach them at the hotel. It seemed that each time I called, they were out. I grew more and more irritated as I waited for them to call back. One day. Two days. Three days went by without a word. When I finally got through, they were surprised to hear from me. Convinced that they had already called us, they were stunned to learn that they hadn't.

"But it's such a nice surprise to hear from you," Mom chirped, as though they'd been living in Israel for thirty years.

This was the last of Herman and Susie's excursions. Although granting them the freedom of this "journey into anguish" was rewarding, seeing their diminished cognizance and competence made it obvious that any long-term travel would be a flagrant temptation of tragedy. Their inability to recognize their own shortcomings made this decision all the more difficult to carry out. They were fully convinced that they could do anything they were able to do fifty years ago, and trying to persuade them otherwise was usually futile.

How difficult it was as a caregiver to convince them that their safety and well-being must often be purchased at the high cost of their dignity and independence. Then again, how satisfying it was not having to deal with the image of Herman and Susie wandering aimlessly in a strange, foreign city.

Postscript

When I was twelve years old, I had my first real travel experience. I had relatives who lived in the Kansas City area and operated a dairy farm for many years. I first visited the farm on a two-week trip with my aunt and uncle, and I was excited because, not only was I about to meet many people for the first time, I also was going to experience my first ride in an airplane.

This was travel, or so I thought.

The next year, I was invited to make the same trip but with a twist: I was to travel solo. My mom and dad put me on the plane in New York, but from there I flew across the country by myself. This time, I was still excited but I also felt a degree of fear that I hadn't before. I remember being thrilled after we stopped in Chicago and took off again into the darkening skies of a summer storm, watching lightning through the window on the way from Chicago to Kansas City.

Those early travel adventures sparked in me a wanderlust that I've had all my life—from job relocation assignments to vacation travel. Seeing that same love of traveling at work in Herman and Susie, even as they entered their nineties, made it all the more difficult to ground them.

4

Time Is
Relatives

I was never really sure what time zone Herman and Susie believed they were in. Asking them to assume the maintenance of a complex technological device like a digital clock would have been comparable to asking a squirrel to lecture on genetic engineering at Harvard. If an appliance was any more complicated than one is likely to find, say, in the home of an Amish minister, they simply would not use it.

Television remote controls, telephones, thermostats, microwave ovens—these were devices they could skillfully operate years ago. Now they not only didn't remember how to use them, but they wouldn't even try.

Their apartment had two television sets, a digital clock/radio and an AM/FM stereo with a cassette player, all of which remained off unless I turned them on. Regardless of when I would set the time on the clock/radio, by the same time the next day they would have changed it again because they simply couldn't believe the time stated was right and were compelled to adjust it by two or three hours in any given direction. Consequently, they stared at each other in disbelief when the living facility where they resided announced that it was time for lunch, and they were still cleaning the breakfast dishes.

The only device they seemed completely uninhibited in using was the speed-dial button on the telephone. As a result, I spent countless hours over the years engaged in conversations like this:

"It's 7:30 on the bedroom clock, but we haven't gotten dinner yet."

"That's because it's only 5:00 P.M. Look at your watch or the kitchen clock."

"Well, the kitchen clock said it was 2:30, so Herman took his afternoon nap. He just woke up and he thinks it's morning. He wants breakfast."

"But it's almost dinnertime."

"He keeps calling down to the kitchen, demanding to know where his breakfast is. He says they're confused."

"They're not confused!" I shout. "He's the one who's confused!"

"He's not right in the head," my mother says. "You'd better come over and take him to the hospital."

The problem was not limited to electronic devices. Although newspapers are hardly the height of technology, Mom and Herman's insistence on saving at least three to five days' worth of papers only stoked the smoldering confusion. Sometimes, Herman would call to tell me that the newspaper he was reading was tomorrow's paper.

"How can I be reading Tuesday's paper when it's only Monday?" he asked with profound gravity.

"If you don't let the housekeeper throw out old papers, then you're bound to pick up one from last week and think it's today's."

He'd think about it for a moment and respond

thoughtfully, "They're late with the lunch again, you know."

Possibly the height of the technological turmoil came when one of them would try to leave a message on our home answering machine. I don't have exact statistics, but I'd estimate that about 75 percent of the time they were completely unaware that they were talking to a machine and not to me.

"He won't talk to me," Mom would tell Herman after several postbeep seconds of complete silence.

"Why won't you talk to us?" Herman would ask my machine, dejected. "If you don't say something, we'll be very upset with you!"

There also were times when they would forsake speed dialing and attempt to reach the outside world (probably to find out why I was still not speaking to them or why *The Price Is Right* had been moved to 2:00 A.M.). I rarely found out about such calls until bill-paying time came around and I wasn't able to figure out how they spent $197.50 to call the Walgreens across the street by routing the call through twelve switchboards in Zurich.

Herman and Susie's adventures with technology provided our family with bittersweet experiences, a lot of laughs and a little bit of irritation. I was often left to wonder how they'd get by if something were to happen to me. Worse, I was frightened by the prospect of what the future holds for me when I'm their age.

Postscript

I have a gold pocket watch that was given to me by my father, which was given to him by his father. I will pass it on to my son, who, down the road, may pass it on to one of his children or to my oldest grandson.

What is this thing we have with watches and time? I have many material possessions that I value but none of them compare to time. After undertaking the care of Susie and Herman, the time that they squandered simply trying to figure out what day it was became my most priceless commodity. Much of the time that I would have used fishing and cruising the Florida Keys, relaxing with friends or even sitting around the house was now spent on repetitive phone calls, trips to the supermarket, visits to the doctor and other countless chores. Even my work time was frequently interrupted, as I was never more than a few feet from a phone.

I sometimes wondered what I would do with the hours I got back after Susie and Herman were gone.

But I didn't have long to do that before the next crisis arose, and I was back on the job again.

5

A Table for Two

It's never easy to watch the elderly struggle with failing health. Often, it is as hard on the significant other as it is on the one who is sick, regardless of the couple's age. The thought of living without your soul mate can conjure some frightening images.

Herman had emergency surgery to correct a severely ruptured bowel that was threatening him with peritonitis, as well as a prostate problem that was in dire need of surgery. Both problems were addressed during a hospital stay, which to call grueling and arduous would be akin to calling the Pacific Ocean wet or the Sears Tower tall. Words are simply inadequate.

Herman spent the better part of his hospital stay fighting with the nurses and pulling out his

IV tubes, to the point where he had to be restrained. After discharge from the hospital, he was admitted to a rehab center for three weeks to help with his recovery. During both stays, my mother was completely confused and had no idea what was going on with Herman. I drove to Miami daily to take her to visit him. On a few weekends, my daughters would take her to visit, but their jobs, children and husbands limited their assistance to the weekends. As a self-employed hotel consultant and commercial Realtor, my schedule was more flexible and I could afford to spend more time making the trips to Miami.

I had no idea that those trips would be the more enjoyable part of Herman's convalescence.

When Herman came home, we employed nurses for two shifts a day to help him bathe, dress, eat and maintain himself. The male nurses were my mother's favorites. The female nurses, however, she held in considerably less regard. When one of the nurses would take Herman into the bathroom to bathe him or help him with his toilet problems, Mom would fly into fits of jealous rage, demanding that they leave her husband alone. Completely unaware—or uncaring—of the general precepts upon which the nursing profession is founded, she insisted that the female nurses provide care for him without actually touching him. If one of them, for some reason, found herself unable to resist putting her hands on Herman, Mom would yell at her until the wanton hussy acquiesced. Mom's behavior got so out of control that several nurses quit. One even called me in tears late one night to say she couldn't take it anymore and was going to leave.

My attempts at speaking with my mother about her behavior were at first met with denial. This line of defense gradually evolved into accusations that the nurses were trying to steal her husband and take money from him. She had no explanation as to why only the female nurses, and not the males, were robbing their patient blind.

Herman recovered from his illness, but my mother's jealousy raged unabated. She constantly accused other women of trying to steal him away from her. She also accused him of going out to meet women in secret in the dining room or lobby. When he spoke to another woman in the elevator, lobby or dining room, my mother would tell the woman to leave her husband alone and not talk to him again. It got so bad that their usual dining-room table, which they shared with two other ladies for lunch and dinner, had to be changed so that Herman and Susie could have their own table for two.

Herman was Susie's anchor. Without him, she would have drifted away like a boat at sea. Knowing that made her all the more jealous of any threat—perceived or real—that might carry him away.

Postscript

Although my mother took care of my father during his illness, such a brief period of time elapsed between his diagnosis and his death that there wasn't a lot of caregiving involved. He went quickly, so Mom had to think more about how she was going to survive without him than how to keep him alive.

Also, Dad was still able to do a lot of things for himself right up until he passed away. He could move around and eat and complete normal day-to-day functions. Even so, my mother took good care of him. I believe I got a lot of my compassion from her, and from my father, who also was a very caring person.

After attending college, I pursued my career in the hotel business, which took me to places like Boston, Washington, D.C., Puerto Rico and Florida. I never moved back to my hometown of New York. For many years after my father passed away, I felt a bit guilty, as though I had abandoned my mother because I was always away. She had her own life and she was very happy. She had friends and a few boyfriends, although she never wanted to remarry until she met Herman.

It wasn't until I saw her fanatical devotion to Herman, and her fear-fueled jealousy over him, that I began to understand: She had lost both my father and me in a brief period of time. Although she was self-sufficient, socially adept and industrious, I imagine there had to be times when she felt terribly alone, with no one to provide emotional support.

Herman was the last great love of her life. She couldn't bear the thought of living without him. In the end, she didn't have to.

6

Open Wide

I had thought that dealing with Mom and Herman's dental needs would be the least of my worries, as Mom wore a partial and needed only an occasional dental check, and Herman, who had a complete set of bridgework, had no need of dental services.

One day, however, one of Herman's nurses told me that his lower plate had somehow broken and that he needed to go to the dentist to see if it could be repaired. I made an appointment for the next afternoon and drove him to the office, with Mom along for the ride, lest he return and be accused of spending his day out carousing with other women. Mom's dementia only added to the anxiety. She rarely remembered why we were making the trip, often wondered whether the appointment was for her or Herman, and usually forgot this information only moments after being told. The added difficulty of having her along, however, was minuscule compared with the furor that leaving her at home would have wrought. (Fortunately, one of my daughters lived near Herman and Susie. As a teacher, her schedule permitted her to help me out with several of the afternoon appointments.)

The dentist examined the broken plate and said that it was not fixable; Herman would need another complete set of dentures. He then took impressions so he could make a mold of Herman's jaw and gums, and we scheduled a return visit for a first fitting the following week. In the meantime, Herman was stuck using only his upper plate. This required a bland diet of eggs, white bread, soups, pound cakes and any other foods that required a minimum of chewing. During the next three weeks, we made several trips to the dentist for fittings. Finally, we got the new teeth and silently thanked the god of bicuspids.

Before leaving the office, the dentist placed

Herman's old set of uppers in a plastic case. The machine that seals teeth in an airtight plastic bag, he told us, was not working. When we got home, I placed the plastic case in Herman's dresser drawer without mentioning it.

Despite a few additional trips to the dentist for fittings, Herman started complaining a few weeks later that his teeth still weren't right and began making rather disparaging remarks concerning the marital status of the dentist's parents. I made yet another appointment with the office, complaining to the receptionist that this situation was unacceptable and must be corrected once and for all, as my fragile mental state—as well as Mom's and several nurses'—hinged on the outcome of Herman's plates.

At the appointed time, we went back to the dentist, and I sent Herman in for his examination while I sat in the waiting room. A few moments later, the dentist called me into the room where Herman sat, leaning back in the chair, his mouth wide open. The dentist scratched his head for a moment, and I braced myself for a protracted medical explanation that would require textbooks, slides and lengthy term papers on the evolution of dentistry since the Middle Ages. *What next?* I wondered. *Does Herman have some bizarre tropical gum blight requiring an emergency airlift to see a specialist in Paris?*

Instead, he proceeded to show me that Herman had his new lower plate and old uppers, solving the problem of Herman's complaints of pain and discomfort. But what had happened to the new uppers, and how did he find the old ones?

It seems that Herman had a habit of wrapping his teeth in a paper napkin when he took them out of his mouth. Somehow—and I sincerely doubt the world's finest investigative minds will ever be able to ascertain precisely how—the new uppers were thrown out. It was back to the dentist for several more visits for another set of uppers.

If any more missing teeth had suddenly turned up in an old suitcase or a long-forgotten storage box in the closet, we were seriously considering the establishment of a denture museum.

Postscript

Confusion is a daily part of a caregiver's existence. What begins as simply misplaced reading glasses or forgetting a commonly used phone number gradually evolves into an inability to maintain even the simplest, most vital aspects of daily living.

Along the way, it is crucial that caregivers find an outlet or a means of escape. The weighty burden of managing the care of a dependent person isn't usually dropped on us all at once. Rather, it is a gradual process that is deceptive because what at first might seem manageable and practical can easily mushroom into disorder and upheaval. On your first day as a caregiver, you may find it inconvenient but acceptable to have missed an important business meeting because your charge forgot to tell you about a doctor's appointment. Six months into your caregiving days, you may lose your temper and start screaming at a loved one over some misplaced dentures.

My fishing boat is my major outlet for recreation and for letting off steam. To me, there's nothing like being ten miles offshore in the ocean, with nothing around but the blue sky and water, just cruising along and trolling for fish. Even though I know I can't be away for long, just having a few hours to myself to do something I love means all the difference in handling the incredible pressure I'm under. I also love bike riding, and I find that the exercise improves my frame of mind and increases my self-control in difficult situations.

I would also recommend that all caregivers do one very important thing: relate your experiences. It helps for any caregiver to have someone to share this all with, whether it's a friend, a spouse, a child, or anyone who'll listen and has some sort of a vested interest in your well-being and sanity. It is especially helpful if the caregiver can relate to someone who has had a similar experience or is knowledgeable enough to offer rational and measured advice. I was fortunate enough to have a very close friend who I had known for about thirty-five years. He offered me a lot of advice and was compassionate and understanding of the problems I was going through with Susie and Herman. When he recently passed away at age seventy-six, I felt a tremendous sense of loss. I often called him to discuss my problems, and he was always there to listen and offer advice, much like an older brother would. He was informed, well-read and well-educated, and he never gave me bad advice. I truly miss his counsel.

At times when there is no one to listen, caregivers can also keep a journal or record their thoughts on a tape recorder. Be open and honest about your feelings, as well as meticulous about recording even small details. As your caregiving days go on, you will be able to look back on mistakes you may have made, or emotions you may have felt, and realize how much you've grown and where you're headed.

Above all, recognize that giving care to someone else doesn't mean you stop caring for yourself.

7

Wired for Emergencies

After attending a posh affair with my wife one evening, we returned home in the tiniest hours of the morning and used the last remaining shards of our energy to slip into bed. About one hour before daylight, the phone rang.

"How do I call the kitchen?" Herman asked.

"The kitchen?" I stammered, still jolted by the sound of the phone at half-past ungodly. "You want to call the kitchen? It's not even light out yet. We only just got home a few hours ago."

Herman giggled as though I'd told him a dirty joke.

"What number do I call to get the kitchen?"

Even in the addled throes of profound sleep deprivation, I realized that trying to enlighten

Herman about the inconvenient timing of his call would be about as productive as threading a needle with my feet. I repeated the number three times and hung up, knowing that getting back to sleep was now going to be impossible.

On other occasions, the ring of the phone had been the herald not of giggles and forgotten phone numbers, but of frightening news. Once, Mom fell down in the lobby, broke her wrist and was sent by ambulance to the hospital. Six months later, Herman was hastening to the dining room, trying as always to be a step ahead of the others, when he slipped (or perhaps was pushed). He tumbled onto my mother, whose five-foot, ninety-six-pound frame crumpled beneath him. He tried to break his fall by putting out his arm, which resulted in a sprained wrist and hand for him, and a badly bruised hip and back for Mom. That phone call came at about 6:00 P.M. and resulted in another anxious trip to a North Miami emergency room.

Fortunately, not all of the calls were accompanied by such dire news. Most were merely annoyances that arrived at the most ill-timed moments possible, usually just before dinner, in the early morning or about thirty to sixty minutes after lunchtime.

Although the morning phone calls usually revolved around the nurses' handling of Herman, sometimes Susie found herself in an empty house and couldn't remember when Herman had left, where he was going, who he was with or when he was scheduled to return. Just as she was preparing a national campaign to plaster his face on every milk carton between Florida and the Yukon, Herman would return from his thirty-minute trip to the bank.

Almost without fail, the afternoon calls meant one thing: They had overslept and missed lunch. Mom liked to take a nap after breakfast and would ask Herman to wake her in an hour. Herman would then fall asleep on the couch while reading the newspaper and they didn't even begin preparing to go to lunch until around noon. By the time they arrived at the dining room an hour or more later, the staff would inform them that lunch was served ninety minutes ago and was now over. Then they would arrive back in their room and call me to complain that the staff was depriving them of food.

"It's okay, we can go out someplace and get a sandwich," Mom would say, oblivious to the fact that they couldn't travel alone. At this point, I would hang up and immediately call the front desk. I would ask that the kitchen put together a few sandwiches for Herman and Susie. They would oblige me, and I was thankful because my options were running low.

Other early afternoon or predinner calls from Mom usually meant that something was wrong with Herman. Sometimes, her diagnosis was simply that Herman was acting up. However, on two occasions when she called, there was really something wrong with Herman. Despite her confusion and inability to remember even the simplest information, Mom always seemed to know that when she got no answer at my home, she could reach me at the office. Both times required my calling the on-premises nurse's office and getting immediate help for Herman. He had had two small strokes in the past year and, thanks to Mom's ability to reach me, we were able to get help for him immediately.

Out-of-town trips required that their calls be forwarded to my cell phone. This greatly limited the amount of time we could plan to be away and made escaping their persistent calls virtually impossible. It was especially challenging to be two thousand miles away and get a call from Mom asking if I could come over to help Herman find his glasses.

Postscript

My mother got into the habit of calling me at least three or four times a day about the slightest Herman-related problem: "I don't know where he's disappeared to," "I don't know what's wrong with this man," "He doesn't make sense when he talks to me."

Herman, on the other hand, rarely called for a specific reason. Sometimes, he'd mumble about something in the newspaper or ask a question, but he no longer had the mental capacity or awareness to say, "I didn't get my dinner," or "The TV isn't working." At times, I couldn't even get out of him what he was calling about. Then I had to call back and ask the aide if he was all right.

In many ways, the convenience of telephones, especially cellular phones, became like a chain around my neck. I was reminded many times each day of my responsibilities. I was called on to make snap decisions, react in emergencies and provide a service. I had considered planning a trip to Europe with my family, but we all knew that, even if we went, we wouldn't feel comfortable about being out of contact from Herman and Susie for that long.

Although my grown children were able to help at times, I was still vexed by the persistent feeling that I was the final decision maker who should be calling the shots in an emergency. As a result, we were always wired for that emergency.

For the constant caregiver, the telephone is both a blessing and a torment. It can be a lifeline that helps us recognize and react instantly to emergencies, but it can also be an anchor that chains us to a never-ending stream of inopportune minutiae that interrupts our lives when we least want it to. The 5:00 A.M. request for the kitchen's phone number was the cost of being on call for the life-threatening crisis.

8

Quest for Keys

The phone rang at 5:30 P.M. and my sub-conscious Caller ID told me who was calling. I had just spoken with them thirty minutes before, so I doubted it was an emergency and wondered if I should let the answering machine get it. I decided to pick up.

Herman was upset because Susie would not give him the keys to their apartment. About three weeks prior, Herman had given his set of keys to the woman at the desk downstairs and asked for another set to be made. For some reason, neither the new set of keys nor the originals materialized. Herman claims that the woman says she lost them, or that she kept them, or that someone did something with them. Despite these fuzzy recollections, one fact remained clear: They had but one set of keys between them.

I probably could have prevented this argument if I had remembered to have another set of keys made. I had considered doing that after discovering that my mother's gold necklace had been taken for the second time, and that an envelope containing $260 in cash was also taken a week later. However, I had been concentrating on suspects, police contacts and changing the locks, and, unfortunately, I hadn't given much consideration to getting an extra set of keys. Now, Herman and Susie were arguing over proprietorship of the sole remaining set of keys.

"I need them in my pocket," he pleaded.

"The key tag has 'Susie' written on it, so they're mine," Mom retorted, "and you can't have them."

Herman claimed to need the keys to take with him when they went out to dinner. Mom countered by saying she wasn't going to dinner, and, therefore, he had no need of keys. I saw my chance to intervene and I took it.

"Go on down and have dinner alone if she refuses to go with you," I told Herman, assuming that she would cave in and go along with him. I realized immediately that I'd jumped in too soon.

Herman said, "I can't go, because she won't give me the keys!" Without the keys, he said, he couldn't get back into the apartment. I came up with another solution: I asked Mom to go to dinner with him.

"Absolutely not," she said.

"Let him lock the door and you carry the keys in your purse," I said.

"No."

"Please?"

"No."

"Mom, yes."

"No."

I recognized that it was time to play hardball and tell Mom that if she wouldn't give Herman the keys, I wouldn't speak to them again and I'd wash my hands of this nonsensical behavior. Sensing that my rising blood pressure and high-pitched tone could spell trouble, she said that she didn't want me to be upset and she was sorry and I shouldn't get involved.

Suddenly, I heard Herman in the background shouting for the keys. At the same time she was shouting, "No!" She also told Herman that he shouldn't call me again, that he could go down to dinner by himself, and that she wouldn't go with him.

With no common ground in sight, I hung up and called the nurse's office, hoping that I could persuade someone to call Herman and Susie and tell them that they needed to go to dinner. No answer. Now I was getting desperate. I waited twenty minutes and called them back, hoping that if no one picked up, they would have just settled the matter and gone to dinner.

"Hello?" Mom answered.

Innocently I asked, "Aren't you late for dinner?"

"Oh my, I didn't realize the time!" she said. "Herman, we better get going or we'll miss dinner. Now, where are those keys again?"

Postscript

Taken individually, many of Herman and Susie's antics seemed amusing—even a little charming—but for the caregiver who has to endure them all day, every day, they can become tedious and taxing. Having the same endless conversations, repeating explanations that you've repeated several times already, reciting instructions over and over again, and quarreling about even the most trivial incidents can bring on fatigue, depression and anger. Caregivers who undertake this assignment without a strong support system risk both their physical and mental well-being.

My wife, Suzanne, was with me throughout my efforts to care for Herman and Susie. She sympathized, listened when I got upset and offered me comfort when I needed it. I shared a lot of my emotions with her, and without her support, I'm not sure I could have endured the hardships. But there were things I didn't share with her because I felt, at times, that I didn't want to burden her with them. It is sometimes too easy for caregivers to unload all their hurt, irritation and resentment on anyone who'll listen, especially family, friends, spouses and partners. However, if burdened caregivers aren't cautious, they can easily make their problems the problems of their sympathizers.

On some occasions, I felt that Suzanne was not as receptive to hearing all my troubles as I might have wanted her to be. She identified with me, even felt sorry for me, but she didn't have the same emotional investment in it. Both her parents passed away more than ten years ago, so she didn't have the experience of caring for very elderly parents. I could actually understand that kind of feeling. It's not a bad thing; it's a human thing. It wasn't necessary for her to have had that experience to relate to it. The important thing was that she listened. Caregivers need to understand that empathy is a double-edged sword: It can mean having sympathy and compassion for another person's situation and feelings, but it can also mean absorbing someone else's problems and making them your own. When caregivers expect their significant others, or anyone for that matter, to absorb, adopt or accept their problems as a way of relieving their burdens, they have crossed the line into codependence.

More simply put, sympathy is not complicity.

9

Money and Medicine

One of the more complicated aspects of caring for my mom and Herman revolved around their insatiable desire for independence. It was the one thing that boosted their self-respect, affirmed their dignity and gave them the incentive to get up each morning. This independence, however, came at a price. Allowing them the freedom to get around on their own, set their own hours and make their own decisions was a process fraught with concern and apprehension for even the most trivial of life's daily exercises. But when it came to life-and-death issues such as money and health, that apprehension was magnified tenfold.

Money was a sensitive issue for us, primarily because Herman had a difficult time counting it and Mom often misplaced it.

Herman had lost his ability to calculate currency. He would go to the bank to cash a check for two hundred dollars and ask for denominations of fifty, ten and five dollars. Standing at the teller's window, he would calculate with pen and paper the amount of each denomination he thought he would need, unaware of the lengthening line of irate bank customers piling up behind him. I had seen him struggle for as long as forty-five minutes at simply breaking down two or three hundred dollars into manageable numbers.

He usually asked the teller to put the money into two or three different envelopes, which he then tucked into the different pockets of his jacket. When Mom was with him, he gave her one or two of the envelopes to store in her purse, in case she needed the money to go shopping. Within a few days, the money was gone and they were astonished by its disappearance. Mom always had a habit of taking things out of her purse and forgetting where she put them. An abundance of the items in her purse were wrapped in paper and carelessly discarded. It is quite likely that she threw away thousands of dollars in cash this way.

At the other end of the spectrum, Herman had taken to hiding money around the apartment: in drawers, cabinets, closets and clothing. By the time he ran out of the money he could locate, he had long since forgotten where he put the surplus cash and would be asking to return to the bank to cash another check. Unfortunately, some of the more unscrupulous help we employed had little trouble locating Herman's hiding places.

As more money began to disappear, I realized that I needed an immediate solution to the problem. I went to the nearest office-supply store and purchased a small cash box with two keys. I explained to Herman and Susie that the box would be used to contain all their cash and that they should only open it to take out a few dollars as needed.

It was still difficult to account for much of the cash. They didn't go out unless I took them and they didn't shop for anything. I paid by check for their personal needs, such as dry cleaning, pharmaceuticals, toiletries and cleaning supplies. Yet, they still had trouble accounting for much of their cash. They claimed that they tipped the help, but that was strictly forbidden and would be grounds for dismissal for anyone caught. Also, these aides were well paid and usually didn't take advantage of their confused patrons.

On the whole, however, the cash box helped solve the problem. Money that once disappeared in two or three days was now around for seven to ten days.

The handling of money was a serious situation for us, but not as dire as the problem with medications. As often as they forgot where they put their money, Herman and Susie forgot either the dosage of their prescription medications or whether they'd taken them at all, despite a daily dispensing system. (Herman was overzealous about refilling the medication dispenser and would often replace a pill once he'd taken it, adding instead of subtracting to the total amount they were to take for a given period.) Under the law, aides could not take their charges' medications with them. The medications must remain in the client's home.

I thought of another simple solution, borrowed entirely from our money problems: I bought a lockable medication box. This way, I reasoned, the nurse's aides could come to the apartment each day and give Herman and Susie their proper dosages. Problem solved, or so I thought. One day, one of the aides went to retrieve medicine from the medication box and found, instead, cash inside. Herman had switched the boxes, inadvertently leading us to the discovery that, because the same manufacturer made both boxes, the keys were interchangeable. Fortunately, my mother had only overdosed on some Tums, instead of her thyroid or bone-strengthening medications.

We then replaced the box with a different model that was padlocked. The nurses carried the keys and dispensed the medications as they were needed. The cash box did not fare as well. Herman and Susie both lost their keys. The box sat in a drawer, empty.

Postscript

One of my most firmly held beliefs is respect for people and their rights. I believe that people have the freedom to express their convictions, whether they be in perfect agreement with mine or completely contrary. I've told my children this often; although it is an old-fashioned principle, it is one that is fundamental to any civilized society. This notion of respect for others extends to the right to live life and end life with dignity. When Herman got confused or did irrational things, it was easy to get impatient, or even angry. It was difficult to understand how an act as simple as making change could be so confounding for anyone but a small child, let alone someone who had lived so long and was once a respected business manager. But it was at times like these that I tried to remember the value of respect and dignity.

Herman was a sweet, likeable and gentle man who I had never known to be anything other than decent and kind since I met him. Knowing that I'd lost my father when he was fifty-six and I was only twenty-four, Herman would sometimes joke with me after he married my mother and say, "Hey, I'm your father now and you have to listen to me." And I'd say, "Of course, Herman. I'll listen because you have become my stepfather." As Herman and I grew closer, he became a surrogate father for me, and it made me happy that I was able to be there for him. When my dad became ill, I wasn't able to or it wasn't necessary for me to be there for him because he had my mother to take care of him. My main concern for Herman was that he be allowed to live and die with respect and dignity, despite the forget-fulness, the mishaps and the confusion. I knew that he, and my own father, would want the same for me.

10

At the Doctor's

L ike many elderly people, Herman and Susie required frequent trips to the doctor's office. Their health was fragile and required diligent care. Mom had been coping with a more advanced stage of dementia than Herman, and also had problems with her thyroid and osteoporosis. Herman had suffered from mild strokes, and as a result he had limited use of his left arm and leg. Given their advanced ages, these ailments seemed mild in comparison to the maladies many seniors endure. Semiannual trips to a physician helped keep their medical problems to a minimum. The trips themselves, however, could be as distressing as the illness they were meant to preclude.

Recently, as we were preparing for a trip to the doctor's office, I resolved that I would try to make the excursion as painless as possible for all of us. I informed the aide that I really needed Herman and Susie in the lobby and ready to go by 10:30 A.M. At 10:10, I called to remind them I was on the way. Herman assured me that they were dressed and waiting. At 10:25, I arrived and called from the lobby to tell them I was waiting for them, reminding them again that we were going to the doctor's office. They said they were on their way down.

Ten minutes went by without a sign of them. I called again. They said they were trying to leave but "Herman had stuff all over the place," and Mom didn't know what he was doing. When I got Herman on the phone, he told me that he couldn't find his keys and was speculating on the possible suspects who might have taken them. I convinced him to leave immediately, to use Mom's keys to lock up, and that we would look for his keys later.

As I began surrendering any hope of making our appointment on time, I discovered that the facility had been having problems with their elevators. Many of the residents were upset because only one elevator was in working condition. The staff had done its best to cope with the problem—for instance, by arranging for open seating in the dining room so that large numbers of residents wouldn't be clogging the elevator while trying to get to dinner all at the same time. However, the changes did little to help the residents who had grown accustomed to following their usual habits. As I waited in the lobby, I watched the single working elevator belch out large groups of irate residents mumbling about the poor service. None of them, however, were Herman and Susie. Desperate, I enlisted the help of the facility's executive director, who commandeered the elevator so that we could get to the fourth floor and fetch the tardy twosome.

It was in the car on the way to the office that Mom asked for the first time, "Where are we going?"

I reminded her again that we were going to the doctor's office for her six-month checkup and, most important, her blood test.

"That's a good idea," she said, satisfied. "Herman should also have a checkup." That, I told her, was also on the agenda.

We entered the doctor's crowded waiting room thirty minutes late and were put at the bottom of the list. Herman and Susie accepted this explanation and we took our seats. About five minutes later, Mom asked, "Why is it we have to wait?" I explained again that we were late for our appointment and had been put at the bottom of the list. Hoping to distract them from the time situation, I gave each of them a magazine to read. Herman seemed to be enjoying his magazine, so I tried talking to Mom about hers by discussing the pictures and articles. We segued into talking about her great-grandchildren and anything else that might keep her mind off the wait.

As the waiting room got emptier and emptier, Mom was getting more and more anxious. She began lambasting the doctor for making us wait and threatened to walk out. When I reminded her again that we were waiting because we had been late, she said that she had prided herself on being punctual her whole life. Regardless, I told her, we were still going to have to wait because they both needed to see the doctor. This line of conversation regenerated about every two minutes.

Almost an hour later, we were called into the examination room, only to find that we'd have to continue waiting while Herman was getting an EKG and blood work done. Mom continued to question why we were kept waiting, incapable of understanding that we had been late.

When the visit finally ended, I took them for lunch at one of their favorite local restaurants, a pancake house, where I calmed myself while they enjoyed their pancakes and eggs. Privately, I reflected on the toll these outings and constant problems had on me physically and mentally. I coped by trying to understand that, should I have the opportunity to live as long as Herman and Susie, I would have to contend with the same difficulties. I remembered how important it was for my own children to see what I was going through with Herman and Susie, so that they, too, would understand this difficult process.

Postscript

We were in Scottsdale, Arizona, horseback riding in the desert, when my horse suddenly threw me, and I cracked some ribs. At the hospital emergency room, suspecting internal injuries, doctors ordered a CAT scan, which revealed a cancerous tumor the size of an orange on my right kidney.

After contacting some friends who were doctors and surgeons, I went through a series of referrals with other specialists. The final recommendation was that the kidney be removed. Before they removed it, however, they wanted to make sure the tumor hadn't spread. Prior to surgery, I had to endure several tests and procedures to be sure that, because of the tumor's size, it had not spread into my bloodstream and other vital organs. The operation was called an abdominal exploratory. Surgeons opened me up, biopsied the tumor, and checked my colon and abdomen for any signs of contamination from the tumor as they awaited the results of the biopsy.

If the cancer had spread, the doctors would have closed me up and sent me home with a dire prognosis. Fortunately, it had been contained to the kidney only, and they removed the affected organ. I spent a few days in the intensive-care unit, during which, according to my wife, Suzanne, there was a period of about eight to twelve hours when I was in bad shape. I went home after five days and was back at work part-time five days after that.

That happened nine years ago, and not a single day has passed that I haven't thanked God for the extra time I've been given on this Earth. I've often thought that I was given this time to care for Mom and Herman, and to be a grandfather to my seven grandchildren, father to my four children, and husband to my wonderful Suzanne.

People have asked me if this experience was frightening, but I'd have to say that I wasn't scared. Perhaps I didn't take it as seriously as other people might, or I just didn't have a bad feeling about it. I actually felt positive about it, thinking, *They're going to take this tumor out and that's going to be the end of it.*

However, I do sometimes wonder about getting ill as I get older. I've been healthy and strong all my life, and I hope I'm able to maintain my current level of fitness. If a severe illness caused me to be dependent on other people to take care of me—be it for the short term or the long term—I would have trouble dealing with that.

As a result, I've changed my lifestyle. I think a lot of that stems not so much from getting older, but getting wiser. I've finally become conscious of dieting and weight, along with cholesterol and blood pressure. I've also slowed down a bit in all my activities, both physical and social. I don't drink anywhere near the amount I used to consume. Alcohol is a depressant and shouldn't be a form of escapism. I ride my bike three or four days a week at 7:00 A.M. for six or seven miles. The exercise helps me start the day with a clear head and gets the cobwebs out. Above all, I've learned that time does enough to steal away our health and vitality. We don't have to help it along.

11

Save That!

A mong Herman and Susie's most baffling behaviors was the gathering and hoarding of things they had no use for. Food was the biggest problem.

They were served three daily meals, including a room-service breakfast delivered promptly at 8:00 A.M. This was a substantial continental breakfast consisting of a serving (for each of them) of two coffees, one serving of milk, one serving of orange juice, two servings of oatmeal, two Danish or coffee cakes and two pieces of fresh fruit. This amounted to quite a lot of food, all of which came packed in individual Styrofoam containers.

For some reason, Herman and Susie found it necessary to keep what they couldn't finish. As a result, an uninitiated visitor who mistakenly opened the refrigerator door was likely to be buried by an avalanche of white containers filled with old coffee, dried-out oatmeal and stale pastries. One of my weekly chores was burrowing into the wall of white and tossing out food they had no intention of ever actually eating.

Lunch and dinner in the dining area were served on china, not Styrofoam, and portions were also more than ample. However, again, when faced with more food than they could consume in one sitting, they immediately set about deciding the question of what to do with the leftovers.

One of Herman's favorite food-salvaging activities involved gathering all the leftover bread, crackers and sweetener packets, wrapping them in napkins and jamming them into his pockets. Nothing was spared, not even the napkins. Mom saved enough napkins to soak Lake Michigan dry.

If they were too full to eat the orange or banana that was usually provided, those items, too, were carefully wrapped in napkins. However, because they sometimes opted not to return to their apartment (choosing instead to hang around the lobby holding hands, watching people walk by or napping), the fruit posed a dilemma when they'd maxed out their available pocket space. Where, oh where, to put the fruit? How about the mailbox?

I still don't know whether this was Herman's idea or Susie's, but I do know one thing for sure: The U.S. Postal Service will not mail fresh fruit. Especially when it has been left in a hot mailbox through the weekend.

Postscript

My parents instilled in me an intense work ethic. I started working when I was a teenager, delivering groceries and dry cleaning, and doing odd jobs. For us, work was meaningful and vital. I could never understand how people could skip work simply because they didn't feel well.

That work ethic was pounded into me, and I've tried to instill it in my children as well. I believe they all got it from watching me over the years and having me show them that there's nothing wrong with hard work as a means of getting what you want.

Susie and Herman were raised in a time when hard work was not as much of an option as it is today. There were no sick days, extended vacations or personal time. Work was a means of survival, and those who didn't work risked their well-being and that of their families. My father worked ten- and twelve-hour days, six days a week, up until his death at age fifty-six. My mother retired, with thirty-five years of service at Bloomingdale's, when she was eighty years old.

It is not hard for me to understand why Herman and Susie hoarded food they would never eat. Although they may not have endured starvation or poverty, they lived during a time when everything you had was the result of hard work, which, in turn, became something to be cherished and valued.

12

The Aid of an Angel

The top priority in providing care for Herman and Susie had always been finding the right person or persons to assist them in their daily living. We had run the gamut of nurse's aides and assisted-living services trying to find the right people. In a year and a half, I went through four agencies, each one of which was, at one time, the "on-the-premises" agency at the adult congregate living facility.

As they aged, Susie and Herman required multiplying degrees of care and personal assistance. They needed help with bathing, dressing, selecting clean clothes, taking medication and ensuring that they were on time for meals. My experience with these agencies was somewhat less than ideal. The best person we were able to find—a

Medicare-assigned home health aide who helped out when Mom broke her wrist and injured her hip in a fall—was one of the most caring and capable I had encountered. But despite my best efforts at hiring her to be Herman and Susie's full-time aide, she said that her plate was already full and declined. So, we continued paying exorbitant fees for the mediocre and indifferent aides often provided by these agencies.

One day, Pam, the efficient and dedicated aide whom I had tried to hire, told us she was available to work as an aide for Herman and Susie. The difference was miraculous. When Herman bathed in the morning, Pam actually made sure that he put soap on the washcloth. She also made sure that he put on all his clothes, including his underwear and socks. Pam helped Mom bathe and dress, and ensured that she took her medication. The beds were made, the clutter was at a minimum, even the Styrofoam jungle that had been left to mutate on the dining-room table and in the refrigerator was a distant memory.

In addition, this angel from above arranged

beauty-salon appointments for Mom and haircut appointments for Herman. Whenever I was scheduled to pick them up for trips to the doctor or shopping, I was sure to find them clean, dressed and in the lobby awaiting my arrival. Pam's devotion to her job and her exceptional ability even made it possible for Herman and Susie to enjoy events that would previously have been impossible.

In the month of March, we celebrated three birthdays in our family. Recently, I had a birthday in that month, my grandson turned four, and Herman was celebrating his ninety-third year of life. We decided on one big party for all these events. In the past, having Herman and Susie over to our house was too much of a chore to be feasible. It required hours of preparation, getting them ready and transporting them to and from the event. Instead, we usually celebrated birthdays at a restaurant near where they lived because it was more convenient for everyone involved. However, on this special occasion, Susie and Herman were able to spend several hours with children, grandchildren and great-grandchildren—all because of Pam's help. My daughter picked them up, and they were dressed, cleaned and ready to go. After hours of picture-taking and merriment, we arranged for a limousine to return them home in grand style. Without Pam, this memorable family event would have been impossible. She was nothing less than a godsend for Herman and Susie. The quality of their lives (and in many ways, mine) improved immensely after her arrival.

Sometimes, prayers are answered.

Postscript

If I had to identify the one thing that makes me outright angry, it would be stupidity. It makes me mad when people do stupid things, and then won't even admit that they've done them, or deny that they've done them. That really sets me off.

As an avid boater for most of my life, it particularly annoys me when people just ignore the rules of the water. Traveling at excessive speeds, they come barreling through no-wake zones, creating big waves that inconvenience and endanger other boaters. Or, they simply don't know what they're doing and ignore basic rules about right-of-way.

Seniors living in communal living facilities face stupidity in the form of incompetence, neglect and outright theft from the people hired to care for them. Some of it is so flagrantly ignorant that you can't believe your eyes. One of the nurse's aides who was working for Herman during his recovery at home asked my mother for a check for five dollars to pay for some skin-care products for Herman. When she got the check, she quickly forged two zeros on it, turning five dollars into five hundred, and deposited the check into her own account. She did the same with several other checks, which I did not discover until I reconciled Susie and Herman's checkbook later that month.

After the discovery, I decided to check on Mom's jewelry, which was quite expensive, and discovered several pieces missing. Thanks to quick action by the police, the aide was arrested a short time later, and the stolen jewelry was recovered in a pawnshop. Because Florida law regarding stolen merchandise recovered in pawnshops requires that the property owner repay the pawnshop the amount of money paid out to the thief, we had to buy back Mom's jewelry. The nursing agency's bonding company repaid the stolen cash with the proof of theft and copies of the police report. The aide was given probation and made restitution to the bonding company, but also lost her license to practice in Florida.

Until Pam came along, I had endured numerous similar incidents of neglect, bungling and blatant disregard for the respect and dignity that all seniors, dependent and otherwise, should receive. As a caregiver, I felt I was fighting a war on two fronts: tending to the needs and demands of Susie and Herman as their bodies and minds degenerated, and also defending them from the seemingly inexhaustible supply of unscrupulous people lining up to steal from them. For caregivers in similar situations, I cannot stress more emphatically the need to find competent and caring nurses and aides. It may seem an insurmountable task to find that one valuable person in a sea of ignorance and ineptitude, but the struggle is well worth the peace of mind you will receive knowing your loved ones are being cared for by someone who cares for them.

13

Emergency Management

On an exceptionally beautiful Sunday afternoon at the park where our family had gathered for the celebration of my grandson's birthday, my cell phone rang at about 5:15. It was Susie and Herman's aide, Pam. Mom had had an asthma attack and was on her way to the emergency room. Mom had occasional attacks of asthma, which could be brought on by a number of different conditions, such as excessive stress or dry air. Because she was susceptible to this ailment, she carried an inhaler in her purse, which helped her breathe when an attack started. Unfortunately, the inhaler was usually anywhere but where it should be when she needed it.

When she found it in her purse, she usually asked Herman, "What is this doing in my purse?"

Herman, depending on his lucidity at the time, would say either, "It's to help you breathe," or "I don't know." When he did explain to Susie that she needed the inhaler to help her breathe, she claimed that she was breathing fine and saw no need to carry this thing around in her purse, at which point she left it on her nightstand with the three others we'd bought to assure that there was always one around.

Despite using the inhaler this Sunday, however, Susie was still having trouble breathing. Pam called 911 and off they went to the hospital. I reached the hospital after a forty-mile drive to find Susie undergoing a battery of tests: EKG, blood work, X rays and more. I explained to the doctor that she had a history of asthma, and he stopped the testing and ordered breathing treatment for her. After a consultation with her personal physician, both doctors agreed that she could go home after the treatment if her lungs had cleared up.

However, Susie's uneasiness increased with every minute she was hospitalized. Because of her failing memory, she needed to be reminded almost constantly about what was happening to her. I decided to pick up Herman, who was not allowed to ride along in the rescue vehicle, and bring him to the hospital. He walked to her bedside and held her hand. She asked him why she was there, and he told her he didn't know. When I explained her condition again, Susie insisted she was fine and demanded to go home.

While this was going on, Herman began acting up, even though he'd been through emergency-room visits before. The shock of seeing a loved one in a potentially life-threatening situation is stressful for anyone, particularly an aged man with diminished faculties. Herman reacted by trying to baby Susie. He kept touching her on the arm, the neck and the feet, almost picking on her in a childlike way. He kept trying to tuck her into the bed by wrapping the blanket around her feet. Susie, however, was not amused. Her admonishments to Herman to stop touching her evolved into shouts demanding that he get away from her.

Finally, I had to have Herman sit on a stool on the other side of the room after the ER doctor,

responding to the noise, ordered that Susie relax
so that the breathing treatment would work effec-
tively. At about 10:30 P.M., we got the okay to
leave, which we tried to do, until we realized
Susie's skirt was missing. The hospital staff told us
that she came in with only a jacket, a blouse,
panties and shoes. As we ushered her into the car
with her blouse covering the hospital gown, she
began asking me to forgive her for disrupting our
Sunday afternoon—a litany she repeated at least
fifty times on the way home, despite my repeating
as many times that she was forgiven. After seeing
them inside safe and sound, I drove back home,
arriving just a few minutes before midnight. I took
a hot shower to unwind, sorry that our Sunday
had been disrupted but very glad that our trip to
the emergency room was a two-way visit.

Postscript

When people reach the advanced years that Herman and Susie did, every health-related incident seems life-threatening while it's happening. During the commotion and confusion that can occur, it gives one pause to think about how aging affects all our lives, from the very young to the very old.

The view from one's middle years is quite different than it is from youth. You not only look back at the joys and mistakes of your younger days, but you also look ahead at what life will be like when you are elderly. This is especially true for middle-aged caregivers, who may be helping their children as they start marriages and careers, but who are also tending to their elderly parents' health-care and living needs.

As we grow older we value different things. As a young man, my worst fear might have been that I couldn't get the car or boat that I wanted. However, as we mature, our value systems change. I think I am like most men and women my age, in that one of my greatest fears is that something bad will happen to a family member, especially to my children or grandchildren. Now, all I want is for them to stay safe and healthy. As they say, the one thing you don't want to do is survive your children. I want them to have their happiness. I've had mine and still have it.

But looking ahead to my own old age is also a source of great apprehension for me. One of the reasons I don't reveal my birthdate is that people tend to put you in a certain category when they know your age. If you say you're forty-five, people tend to assume you're a baby boomer; if you're fifty-five, they assume you've received your AARP membership card. If you say you're sixty-five, then you're an old man ready for retirement. That we are categorized by our age has always been a problem for me. If people don't have a number in mind when they consider you, then they can't necessarily categorize you as a young man, a middle-aged man, an old man or a doddering old fool.

We've all encountered people who are in their fifties and act like they're ready for the retirement home, and we've seen people in their eighties doing things most thirty-year-olds wouldn't consider. Age, for me, is not a number; it is a state of mind. People who do know my age tell me that I look young for it, but that doesn't affect me positively or negatively. We may live in a young world, but I don't feel old, regardless of my age. I can do just about everything I used to be able to do.

14

A Final Word

On April 15, 1999, Susie suffered a stroke as she was eating dinner at the facility where she and Herman lived. Paramedics performed CPR and rushed her to the hospital. The next day, when she showed no signs of recovery, the doctors took her off the respirator and moved her to a hospice room in accordance with her living will. She died there a short time later.

We held a small funeral service for immediate family and some of Mom's friends. We acceded to her wishes to be cremated. Herman was very much in shock and could not understand why this had happened. He spent a long time at the casket talking to her but could not accept the fact that she was gone. He told people that "Susie is away," or "She's not here right now."

About a year after her passing, we purchased a niche at a mausoleum near us and, again, according to her wishes, placed her in the niche with my father's ashes—which she had kept with her all these thirty-five years since his passing—so that they could be together again. Also as they had requested, I purchased a cemetery plot for Herman at the same cemetery, so that the three could be close to one another.

After Susie passed away, Herman's condition went slowly downhill, both mentally and physically. He didn't care what would happen to him after he was gone, and he had trouble accepting the loss and understanding why Susie was gone. His incontinence, decaying memory and medical problems were a constant challenge for us in continuing his care, the same as when Susie was alive. Despite my encouragement, he no longer had interest in passions he cherished for his entire life: painting, chess and music.

At the same time, Herman became closer to the rest of our family. Our children and grandchildren adored him, and he became a late-in-life stepfather for me. I lost my real dad in 1963 but got a new one in 1995, someone whose caring and genial nature brightened the last four years of my mother's life. When I visited Herman, he clapped his hands and was effusive in his happiness to see me.

Just before Mom and Herman married, she asked me to promise her that I would continue to take care of Herman if she passed away first. I made her that promise and I kept it. It's strange, though; long before she passed away, I became quite close to Herman, as a surrogate father, and would have taken on the responsibility of taking care of him without her asking. At the time, I wasn't aware of that, but in all good conscience, what choice did I have? When asked, he always said he had no relatives and only a few friends and some distant relatives on his first wife's side of the family.

In a way, it was a blessing to have Herman to take care of after Susie died. Although taking care of two of them was one of the most difficult things I've ever done, Herman alone was not as much of a burden. He was a kind, decent, sweet person, and I wanted to be able to do anything I could to make him as comfortable as possible; that was my primary goal. I don't think anyone should live in misery. Mom and Herman made arrangements (Mom prior to marriage, and then jointly with Herman after marriage) through an irrevocable family trust, naming me as trustee to handle their assets so they could continue to live in the lifestyle in which they had been living, no matter the cost for aides, medicine, etc.

Although my mother's passing was one of the saddest moments of my life, the time and manner of her passing was not a tragedy. She was ninety-two years old and she went quickly, which was something she had always wished for. She didn't want to linger with a terrible disease or with tubes in her arms and machines keeping her alive. She got her wish, and my family and I, although we lost someone we loved and were very close with—especially over the last seven to eight years of her life—had the opportunity to spend a lot of time with her in the final years. I am grateful for that time. I was still a young man when my father passed away, and, at the time, I was not able to fully appreciate the long-term effects of losing him.

There have been a few times in my life when I've been disappointed in my decisions. When I married the first time, my wife and I eloped without telling anyone our plans. It was a big disappointment to my parents, especially to my father. My father didn't feel that I was ready for marriage because I was too young. Rather than argue with him and try to make him come to a wedding he was against, we sneaked off together and then told them the next day that we'd gotten married. It was a shock to both my parents, who I always felt were disappointed, both in my decision to rush into a marriage we were not ready for and my method of doing it. My father passed away less than seven months later.

Since that time, I've tried to remember how each of our decisions—however trivial they may seem at the time we make them—can have a profound impact on the lives of others. I have always kept this in mind as I tried to help Susie and Herman in their final difficult days, and I will continue to do so as I endeavor to help friends and family in the future. I'm thankful that my decision to move Susie out of the big city of New York to South Florida—and then to let her move into a facility that was far enough from our home to be an inconvenience—ultimately led to her finding Herman. I will always cherish the memory of Herman and Susie holding hands wherever they found themselves. At a time when their faculties had almost completely failed them, they found in each other the seeds of renewal. They were, for each other, anchors in the storm of confusion and chaos that ruled the final years of their lives. Such a blessing is something everyone should experience, regardless of age.

The memory of my parents' marriage is also a comfort to me. They were devoted to each other, loved each other, and taught me the value of hard work and self-honesty, something I've tried to instill in my own children. I also have wonderful memories of my own life that I hope will last until my final days: memories of times good, bad, sad and happy; marriages; divorces; the births of children and grandchildren; high-school days; serving in the army and the experience of entering manhood; playing football and baseball; spending time on my boat; and living out West at my aunt and uncle's farm. So many memories. Maybe those are the most prized possessions we will ever have.

ABOUT THE AUTHOR

Since graduating from college, where he majored in hotel administration, L. B. Smith's entire professional career has been in the hotel business. From his introduction into the hotel industry with Hilton Hotels, Sheraton and Holiday Inn, he held various positions, from general manager to vice president of sales and marketing. He has been president of Hospitality Specialists, Inc., a hotel-consulting company, since 1996.

Three years ago, Smith's close friend, Gary Seidler, who thought Smith's stories about his personal experiences as a caregiver to his mother and stepfather would provide insight and assistance to the many baby boomers in the same situation, encouraged Smith to put these stories on paper. The result is *Susie & Herman*, a memoir he hoped would capture the experience realistically, but with humor and empathy, too.

Smith, a native New Yorker who now lives in Boca Raton, Florida, has been married to the beautiful Mary Suzanne for the past twenty-three years, and between them (from previous marriages) they have four wonderful children and seven grandchildren.